KETO DIET

FOR WOMEN AFTER 50

Reboot your metabolism and burn the fat with quick, easy, and delectable Recipes for Busy Lifestyle

By Matilda Fox

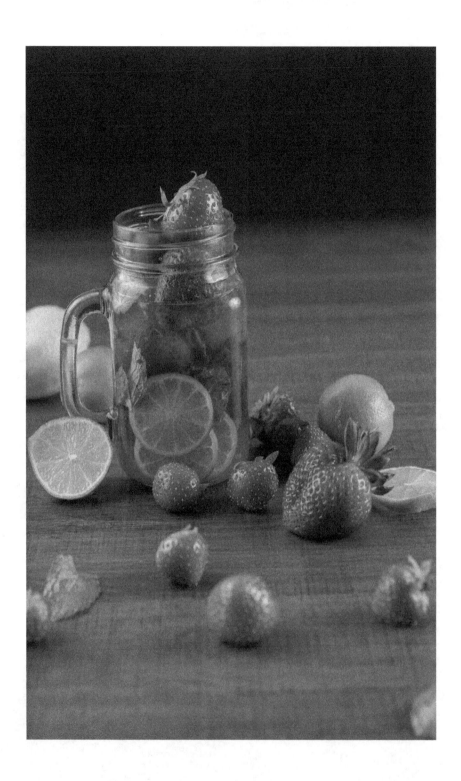

The information in the following pages is broadly considered a truthful and accurate account of facts and as such, any inattention, use, or misuse of the information in question by the reader will render any resulting actions solely under their purview. There are no scenarios in which the publisher or the original author of this work can be in any fashion deemed liable for any hardship or damages that may befall them after undertaking information described herein.

Additionally, the information in the following pages is intended only for informational purposes and should thus be thought of as universal. As befitting its nature, it is presented without assurance regarding its prolonged validity or interim quality. Trademarks that are mentioned are done without written consent and can in no way be considered an endorsement from the trademark holder.

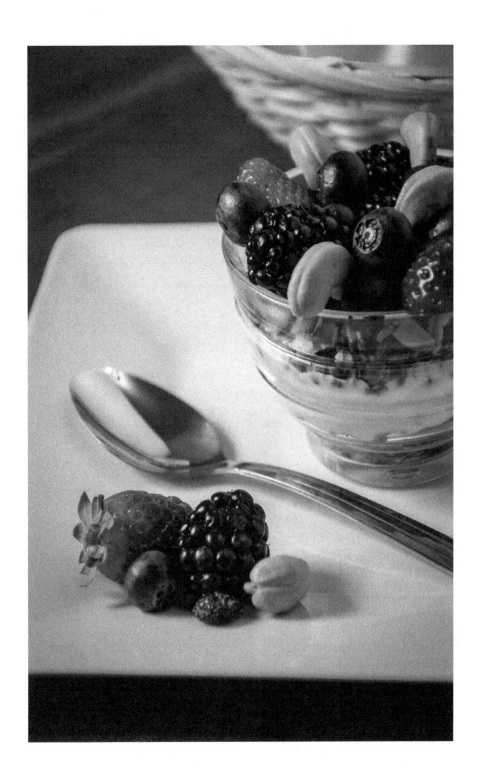

Table of contents

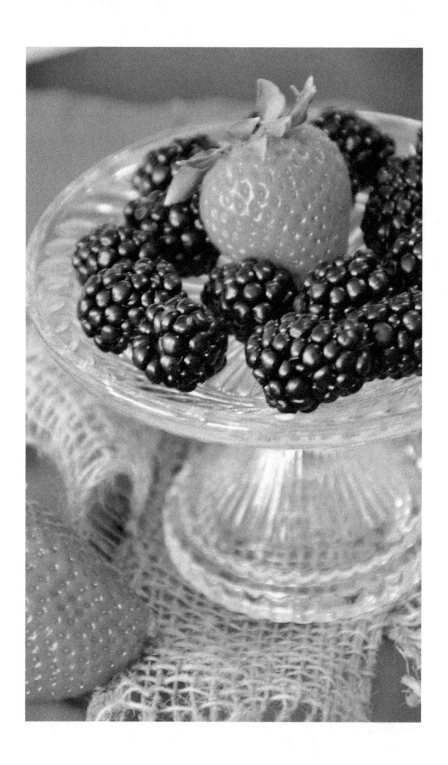

Introduction

Women go through so much in life, don't we? From growing up, discovering the joys of life, pursuing a promising career, becoming a mother, there is so much that changes within such a short period.

While that is a part of life, what anyone would genuinely try and avoid would be putting on excessive weight that we carry around like unneeded luggage. It is embarrassing, it is distracting, and it is causing quite a few internal issues.

If you thought the biggest hurdle you will face when you hit 50 is a big belly, think again. It isn't the only problem we face. While some would say that having a generous belly is the biggest problem, we firmly believe that there are more serious issues to worry about than that. When it comes to women, well, things aren't looking good.

Our bodies, since birth, continuously change. Most of these changes do not harm us and are only natural. However, once we enter into our 50s, things are a lot different. Now, any changes within our body will directly affect how we perform, operate, and work. If we were to keep these changes unchecked and pay no close attention, things would take a worse turn.

Most of these issues will remain the same for men; however, due to our bodies' chemistry and differences, both internal and external, both would face a variety of issues exclusive to their gender. There are a few ways we can avoid these issues. Some of these ways require you to go back in time, start working out from a very young age, control your diet, and change your habits. That is the stuff of science fiction and hence is out of the equation.

Other ways would include visiting a doctor and getting pills and energy boosters to feel better while taking more pills to fight diabetes, high blood pressure, and other health issues. This way is not just hectic but far too complicated as well.

For a very long time, the only other way was to avoid worrying too much and hope that life would fix issues itself, and that never ended well for many. People have then left with worry and a gap that nothing was able to fill. In comes ketogenic diet. Call it a need of the hour, a savior in disguise, or anything you like. The fact remains that this is proving to be a popular option that is not only delivering results but is also helping millions to maintain a healthy lifestyle and reverse some of the damage their bodies have suffered.

Numerous studies have supported the idea that keto diets are far more effective for older men and women than the younger folks. With so much to look forward to and so little to sacrifice, it does make sense to state that Keto is essentially becoming your permanent way of life once you hit 50. But why is that? Why do we proclaim Keto as an important lifestyle choice for women above 50?

The answer to this involves some explanation; as a woman, you have likely experienced significant differences in how you must diet compared to how men can diet. Women tend to have a harder time losing weight because of their different hormones and how their bodies break down fats. Another factor to consider is your age group. As the body ages, it is important to be more attentive to how you care for yourself. Aging bodies start to experience problems more quickly, which can be avoided with the proper diet and exercise plan. Keto works well for women of all ages, and this is because of how it communicates with the body. No matter how fit your body is right now or how much weight you need or want to lose, Keto will change the way that your body metabolizes, giving you a very personalized experience.

When starting your Keto diet, you should not be thinking about extremes because that isn't what Keto should be about. You should be able to place your body into ketosis without feeling terrible in the process. One of the biggest guidelines to follow while starting your Keto journey is to listen to your body regularly. If you ever think that you are starving or simply unfulfilled, you will likely have to modify the way you are eating because it isn't reaching ketosis properly. It is not an overnight journey, so you need to remember to be patient with yourself and your body. Adapting to a Keto diet takes a bit of transition time and a lot of awareness.

The health benefits of the Keto diet are not different for men or women, but the speed at which they are reached does differ. As mentioned, women's bodies are a lot different when it comes to burning fats and losing weight. For example, by design, women have at least 10% more body fat than men. No matter how fit you are, this is just an aspect of being a woman you must consider. Don't be hard on yourself if you notice that it seems like men can lose weight easier — that's because they can! What women have in additional body fat, men typically have the same in muscle mass. It is why men tend to see faster external results. That added muscle mass means that their metabolism rates are higher. That increased metabolism means that fat and energy get burned more quickly. When you are on Keto, though, the internal change is happening right away.

Your metabolism is unique, but it will also be slower than a man's by nature. Since muscle can burn more calories than fat, the weight seems to fall off men, giving them the ability to reach muscle growth quickly. It should not be something that holds you back from starting your Keto journey. As long as you keep these realistic bodily factors in mind, you won't be left wondering why it takes you a little longer to start losing weight. This point will come for you, but it will take a bit more of a process you must be committed to following through with.

A woman can experience another unique condition, but a man cannot be PCOS or Polycystic Ovary Syndrome, a hormonal imbalance that causes cysts' development. These cysts can cause pain, interfere with normal reproductive function, and burst in extreme and dangerous cases. PCOS is very common among women, affecting up to 10% of the entire female population. Surprisingly, most women are not even aware that they have the condition. Around 70% of women have PCOS, which is undiagnosed. This condition can cause a significant hormonal imbalance, therefore affecting your metabolism. It can also inevitably lead to weight gain, making it even harder to see results while following diet plans. To stay on top of your health, you must make sure that you are going to the gynecologist regularly.

Menopause is another reality that must be faced by women, especially as we age. Most women begin the process of menopause in their mid-40s. Men do not go through menopause, so they are spared from another condition that causes slower metabolism and weight gain. When you start menopause, it is easy to gain weight and lose muscle. Once menopause begins, most women lose muscle faster and conversely gain weight, despite dieting and exercise regimens. Keto can, therefore, be the right diet plan for you. Regardless of what your body is doing naturally, via processes like menopause, your internal systems are still going to be making the switch from running on carbs to deriving energy from fats. When the body begins to run on fats successfully, you have an automatic fuel reserve waiting to be burned. It will take time for your body to do this. However, when it does, you will eat fewer calories and still feel full because your body knows to take energy from the fat you already have. It will become automatic. However, it is a process that requires some patience, but being aware of what is going on with your body can help you stay motivated while on Keto.

Because a Keto diet reduces the amount of sugar you are consuming, it naturally lowers insulin in your bloodstream. It can have amazing effects on any existing PCOS and fertility issues and menopausal symptoms and conditions like pre-diabetes and Type 2 diabetes. Once your body adjusts to a Keto diet, you are overcoming the naturally in place that can prevent you from losing weight and getting healthy. Even if you placed your body on a strict diet, if it isn't getting rid of sugars properly, you likely aren't going to see the same results you will when you try Keto. It is a big reason why Keto can be so beneficial for women.

For women over 50, there are guidelines to follow when you start your Keto diet. As long as you follow the method properly and listen to what your body truly needs, you should have no more problems than men do while following the plan. What you will have are more obstacles to overcome, but you can do it. Remember that plenty of women successfully follow a Keto diet and see great results. Use these women as inspiration for how you anticipate your journey to go. When it seems impossible, remember what you have working against you, but more importantly, what you have working for you. Your body is designed to go into ketogenesis more than designed to store fat by overeating carbs. Use this as inspiration or motivation to keep pushing you ahead. Keto is a valid option for you, and the results will prove this, especially if you are over the age of 50.

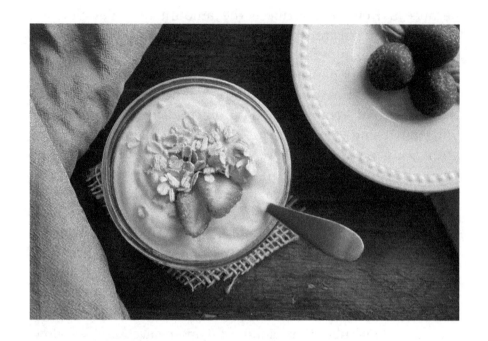

Chapter. 1

Breakfast

1. Scrambled Eggs in A Cup

Preparation time: 15 minutes

Cooking time: 3 minutes

Servings: 3

Ingredients:

- 2 eggs

- 2 tbsp cream to beat
- salt and pepper
- 1 tbsp Butter

Directions:

1. Grease a large bowl using soft butter. Whisk the eggs plus the cream, then fill the cup to a maximum of two thirds, as the eggs will gain volume when cooked.
2. Put a bit of salt and freshly ground black pepper or cayenne.
3. Cook in the microwave at maximum power for 1-2 minutes (700 watts). Stir and microwave another minute. Keep in mind that the eggs are still made after removing them from the heat, so do not overdo them.
4. Remove and add a little butter. Allow cooling for one minute.

Nutrition:

Calories: 107

Carbs: 1g

Fat: 7g

Protein: 7g

2. Ketogenic Frittata of Goat Cheese and Mushrooms

Preparation time: 15 minutes

Cooking time: 22 minutes

Servings: 4

Ingredients:

Frittata:

- 150 g mushrooms
- 75 g fresh spinach
- 50 g chives
- 50 g butter
- 6 eggs
- 110 g goat cheese
- Salt and ground black pepper
- 150 g green leafy vegetables
- 2 tbsp olive oil
- Salt and ground black pepper

Directions:

1. Prepare to preheat the oven to 175 ° C (350 ° F).
2. Grate or crumble the cheese and mix in a bowl with the eggs—salt and pepper to taste.
3. Cut the mushrooms into small pieces. Chop the chives.
4. Melt the butter over medium heat in a pan suitable for the oven and fry the mushrooms and onions for 5-10 minutes or until golden brown.

5. Put the spinach in the pan and fry for another 1-2 minutes. Pepper. Pour the egg mixture into the pan—Bake for about 20 minutes or until browned and firm in the middle.

6. Serve with green leafy vegetables and olive oil.

Nutrition:

Calories: 168

Carbs: 21g

Fat: 4g

Protein: 12g

3. Vegan Scrambled Eggs with Silk Tofu

Preparation time: 15 minutes

Cooking time: 20 minutes

Servings: 3

Ingredients:

- 300 g silken tofu
- 100 g Tofu, tight
- 30 g Nutri-Plus Protein Powder Neutral
- 1 small onion
- A good pinch Kala namak
- Salt, pepper, turmeric
- Fresh chives
- 1-2 tbsp neutral vegetable oil

Directions:

1. Put the silk tofu, the protein powder, turmeric, Kala Namak, salt, and pepper in a blender jar and mix well with the blender.
2. Now crumb the firm tofu, cut the onion into small cubes, and put them under the silk tofu mixture.
3. Warm some oil in a pan, then put the mass for the vegan scrambled egg. Slowly set it to a medium level and stir again and again.
4. Give the scrambled eggs some time; it takes a little longer than the original! But the wait is worth it.

5. Once the desired consistency is achieved, you can fold some fresh chives and enjoy your vegan scrambled eggs.

Nutrition:

Calories: 102

Carbs: 3g

Fat: 0g

Protein: 12g

4. Low Carb Beef Roll

Preparation time: 15 minutes

Cooking time: 60 minutes

Servings: 4

Ingredients:

- 900 g ground beef
- 1/2 tsp fine Himalayan salt
- tsp black pepper
- 1/4 cup yeast
- large eggs
- tbsp avocado oil
- 1 tbsp lemon zest
- 1/4 cup chopped parsley
- 1/4 cup chopped fresh oregano
- cloves of garlic

Directions:

1. Preheat the oven to 204 degrees.
2. Mix the ground beef, salt, black pepper, and nutritional yeast in a large bowl.
3. Beat the eggs, butter, herbs, and garlic in a blender or food processor. Beat until eggs begin to froth, and then add chopped herbs, lemon zest, and garlic.
4. Add the egg mixture to the minced meat and mix. Pour the meat mixture into a small 8 x 4-inch dish—smooth well.

5. Arrange on the middle rack and bake for 50-60 minutes, until the top turns golden brown.
6. Carefully remove from the oven and tilt the mold over the sink to drain all the liquid. Allow cooling for 5-10 minutes before slicing. Garnish with fresh lemon and serve.

Nutrition:

Calories: 86

Carbs: 3g

Fat: 4g

Protein: 8g

5. Crispy Ginger Mackerel with Vegetables

Preparation time: 15 minutes

Cooking time: 30 minutes

Servings: 4

Ingredients:

Marinade:

- 1 tbsp grated ginger
- 1 tbsp lemon juice
- 1 tbsp olive oil
- 1 tbsp coconut amino acids
- Salt and pepper to taste

Fish:

- 2 (about 226 g) boneless mackerel filet
- 28 g almonds
- ½ cup broccoli
- 1 tbsp oils
- ½ small yellow onion
- 1/3 cup diced red bell pepper
- 1 small sun-dried tomatoes (chopped)
- 1 tbsp mashed avocado

Directions:

1. Preheat the oven to 204 ° C. Place a baking sheet on parchment paper or foil.
2. Combine grated ginger, lemon juice, olive oil, coconut amino acids, and a little salt and

pepper. Grate the mackerel fillet with half the marinade.

3. Place the fillet on a baking sheet with the skin up. Bake for 12-15 minutes or until the skin becomes crisp.
4. Place the almonds on a separate baking sheet. Cook for 5-6 minutes or until the nuts turn brown. Remove from the oven and cool before chopping.
5. Lightly steam the broccoli until it begins to soften, but becomes soft. Cut into pieces. Warm the pan over medium heat, then add the oil and let it melt. Sauté the onions and peppers until they are soft.
6. Add broccoli and sun-dried tomatoes, and continue cooking until they heat up. Turn off the heat, then mix with the rest of the dressing and roasted almonds. Serve with the avocado smoothie.

Nutrition:

Calories: 115

Carbs: 4g

Fat: 8g

Protein: 7g

6. Spinach Egg Casserole

Preparation time: 15 minutes

Cooking time: 30 minutes

Servings: 5

Ingredients:

- 283.5 g spinach
- ¼ chopped onion
- 1 minced garlic
- 56.7 g cream cheese
- 59.5 ml buttercream
- 1 tbsp butter
- 1/8 tsp ground nutmeg
- eggs
- Salt and pepper to taste
- 1 tbsp grated Parmesan cheese

Directions:

1. Boil water, then adds salt and spinach and simmer for 1 minute in a pan. Drain the spinach, squeeze, chop and set aside.
2. Warm the oil in a pan, add chopped onion and garlic, and cook for 3 minutes or until it becomes aromatic. Add cream cheese and heavy cream, and cook until smooth.
3. Add chopped spinach and cook for 10 minutes— season with nutmeg, salt, and pepper.

4. Preheat the oven to 204 degrees. Put the spinach your baking dish, then make small indentations with the back of the spoon.
5. Break into each hole in the egg. Bake for up to 15 minutes or until egg whites is cooked.
6. Season the casserole with salt and pepper. Serve sprinkled with grated Parmesan cheese.

Nutrition:

Calories: 110

Carbs: 8g

Fat: 5g

Protein: 8g

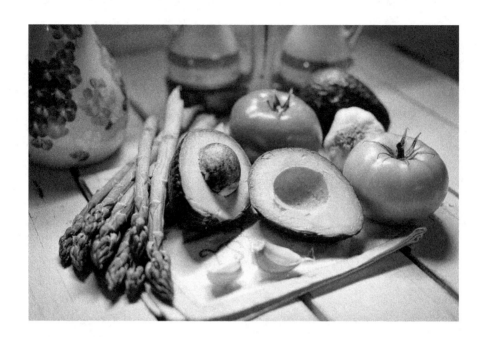

Chapter 2

Lunch

7. Cheesy Buffalo Chicken Lettuce Wraps

Preparation time: 15 minutes

Cooking time: 15 minutes

Servings: 4

Ingredients:

- 1 cup chicken broth (low-sodium)

- 1-ounce cream cheese
- 1/2 cup cheese (cheddar), shredded
- 3/4 cup buffalo sauce
- Blue cheese, crumbled
- Preferred chicken seasoning to taste
- 1 green onion, chopped
- 1 tablespoon Greek yogurt (plain)
- 2 chicken breasts (skinless)
- 4 slices romaine lettuce
- Pepper & salt to taste

Directions:

1. Put the chicken and broth in the IP. Secure the lid and place the pressure valve to seal the position. Set to MANUAL HIGH PRESSURE for 10 minutes.
2. Transfer the chicken to a slicing board. Shred using 2 forks or a knife.
3. Remove the cooking liquid from the pot. Set the IP to SAUTÉ. Add the shredded meat. Add the cream cheese, buffalo sauce, cheddar, yogurt, pepper, salt, and chicken seasoning. Stir to mix.
4. Cook within 2 to 3 minutes or till the cheese is melted. Put the mixture on lettuce wraps. Top with crumbled blue cheese and green onions.

Nutrition:

Calories: 215

Carbs: 2.3g

Protein: 31.5g

Fats: 8.8g

8. Stuffed Avocado

Preparation time: 15 minutes

Cooking time: 0 minutes

Servings: 2

Ingredients:

- 1 large avocado, halved and pitted
- 3 tbsp. mayonnaise
- 2 tbsp. fresh lemon juice
- Salt and black pepper, to taste
- 1 (5-ounce) can water-packed tuna, drained and flaked
- 1 tbsp. onion, chopped finely

Directions:

1. Carefully remove abut about 2–3 tablespoons of flesh from each avocado half. Arrange the avocado halves onto a platter and drizzle each with 1 teaspoon of lemon juice.
2. Chop the avocado flesh and transfer it into a bowl. In the avocado flesh bowl, add tuna, mayonnaise, onion, remaining lemon juice, salt, and black pepper, and stir to combine.
3. Divide the tuna mixture into both avocado halves evenly. Serve immediately.

Nutrition:

Calories: 396

Carbs: 8g

Protein: 19.9g

Fats: 32.3g

9. Keto Crab Cakes

Preparation time: 15 minutes

Cooking time: 10 minutes

Servings: 6

Ingredients:

- 12 oz crabmeat
- ¼ teaspoon salt
- 1 teaspoon chili powder
- 1 teaspoon ground white pepper
- 1 egg
- 1 tablespoon almond flour
- 1 tablespoon butter
- 1 tablespoon chives

Directions:

1. Chop the crab meat into tiny pieces. Put the chopped crabmeat in the bowl. Sprinkle the crabmeat with the salt, chili powder, ground white pepper, and chives.
2. Stir the mixture gently with the help of the spoon. Then beat the egg in the crabmeat. Add almond flour and stir it carefully. When you get the smooth texture of the seafood – the mixture is done.
3. Preheat the air fryer to 400 F. Take 2 spoons and place the small amount of the crabmeat mixture in one of them. Cover it with the second spoon and make the crab cake.

4. Toss the butter in the air fryer and melt it.
   Transfer the crab cakes to the air fryer and cook
   them for 10 minutes. Turn the crab cakes into
   another side after 5 minutes of cooking.
5. When the dish is cooked – chill them gently.
   Enjoy!

Nutrition:

Calories: 107

Carbs: 2.6g

Protein: 9.1g

Fats: 6.1g

10. Beef Satay and Peanut Sauce

Preparation Time: 30 Minutes

Cooking Time: 10 Minutes

Servings: 4

Ingredients:

Beef Satay & Marinade:

- 1/2 teaspoon of coriander, ground
- 2 tablespoons of honey
- 2 tablespoons of Tamari soy sauce
- 2 tablespoons of fish sauce
- 1 pound of flank steak

Thai Peanut Sauce:

- 1/2 teaspoon of Thai red curry paste
- 1 tablespoon of honey
- 1-2 teaspoons of Chile garlic sauce
- 1/3 cup of canned full-fat coconut milk
- 1/4 cup of peanut butter, smooth

Extras:

- Foil
- Bamboo skewers soaked in water for several hours
- 1 tablespoon of olive oil to oil meat before grilling

Directions:

1. Make the beef satay by cutting the steak into 1 1/2inch slice, ensuring that the meat's grain is going lengthwise along strips.
2. Put the meat onto the skewers making sure that you leave a long handle to enable you to hold as you eat the meat.
3. In a baking dish, combine well honey, soy sauce, fish sauce, and the beef, then mix well to ensure that the beef is well coated.
4. Drizzle some coriander on the meat, rub it, and then leave the meat to marinate for around 15-20 minutes.
5. In the meantime, shake well the coconut milk and preheat the grill.
6. For the peanut sauce, warm the peanut butter in a small bowl in a microwave; warm for a couple of seconds, then add in red curry paste, honey, and garlic sauce.
7. Using a whisk, slowly mix in the coconut milk to the mixture, frequently stirring as you add it in.
8. Add around one tablespoon of olive oil on top of the beef and rub it in to ensure the beef is well coated.

9. Fold some foil in half and place under the skewer handles as you cook the meat on the grill.

10. Remove meat from marinade and lay them on the grill, ensuring you put a foil under the skewer handles.

11. Grill, both sides of the beef until well-cooked, then serve with the peanut butter sauce or any salad.

Nutrition:

Calories: 296

Carbs: 12g

Fat: 17g

Protein: 0g

11. Mini Meatloaves

Preparation Time: 5 Minutes

Cooking Time: 30 Minutes

Servings: 12

Ingredients:

- 1 1/2 tablespoons of Dijon mustard
- 3 cloves of peeled and minced garlic
- 1 teaspoon of dry thyme
- 2 loosely packed cups of finely chopped spinach
- 1/2 cup of carrots, grated
- 2 cups of finely chopped mushrooms
- 1 peeled and finely chopped medium onion
- 2 large pastured eggs
- 1 teaspoon of ground black pepper
- 1 1/2 teaspoons of sea salt
- 2 pounds of grass-fed pork

Directions:

1. Prepare the oven to around 350 degrees, then in a mixing bowl, mix all the ingredients.
2. With clean hands, combine well the ingredients until everything is blended.

3. Divide equally the mixture among 12 muffins holes, then bake for about 25-30 minutes until the meat is well done.
4. Serve warm with salad or cauliflower rice, then place the leftovers in a fridge; this can remain fresh for up to 5 days.

Nutrition:

Calories: 168

Carbs: 6g

Fat: 6g

Protein: 20g

12. Greek Meatball Salad

Preparation Time: 10 Minutes

Cooking Time: 20 Minutes

Servings: 4

Ingredients:

For the salad:

- 1/4 cup of parsley leaf, chopped
- 1 lemon, sliced into wedges
- A few lettuce leaves for serving
- 1 tomato, cut into wedges

For the meatballs:

- 4 tablespoons (60 ml) olive oil
- Pepper and Salt
- 2 cloves of peeled and minced garlic
- A large handful of finely chopped mint, about ¼ cup
- 2 teaspoons /2 grams of dried Oregano
- 1 pound/ 450 grams of ground lamb

Directions:

1. Prepare to preheat the oven to about 350 degrees F, then in a mixing bowl, mix pepper, salt, garlic, mint, dried oregano, and lamb.
2. Make small balls from the lamb mixture, put some olive oil in a skillet, and sauté the meatballs in batches until they turn brown.

3. Remove, then put on a baking tray coated with some parchment paper, then bake the meatballs in the oven for around 10 minutes to make sure that the meatballs are well cooked in the middle.
4. Serve with lettuce, and tomato wedges, squeeze some lemon juice from the lemon on top, and garnish with parsley.

Nutrition:

Calories: 440

Carbs: 34g

Fat: 13g

Protein: 42g

13. Low Carb Chicken Philly Cheesesteak

Preparation time: 10 minutes

Cooking time: 15 minutes

Servings: 3

Ingredients:

- 3 slices of provolone cheese
- 1/2 teaspoon of minced garlic
- 1/2 cup of bell pepper, diced, fresh or frozen
- 1/2 cup diced onion, fresh or frozen
- 2 teaspoons of olive oil, divided
- 1 dash of ground pepper
- 1/2 teaspoon of garlic powder
- 1/2 teaspoon of onion powder
- 2 tablespoons of Worcestershire sauce
- 10 ounces or about 2 boneless chicken breasts

Directions:

1. Cut the chicken into very thin slices, then place it in a freezer for a few minutes to make it easier to make this recipe.
2. Put the chicken in a bowl and add in Worcestershire sauce, onion powder, garlic powder, and pepper; toss the chicken to the coat.
3. In an ovenproof pan, put one teaspoon of olive oil, add in the chicken, and cook for around 5 minutes or turn brown.

4. Rotate the chicken pieces over and cook for another 2-3 minutes, until brown. Remove from the pan.
5. Put the leftover olive oil in the same pan, then add garlic, pepper, and onions. Cook while constantly stirring for about 2-3 minutes until they are hot and soft.
6. Reduce the heat and put the chicken pieces back into the pan; stir to combine everything.
7. Put the cheese on top and cover with a lid for another 2-3 minutes until the cheese melts. Serve in bowls and enjoy.

Nutrition:

Calories: 263

Carbs: 5g

Fat: 13g

Protein: 27g

14. Broccoli Soup with Turmeric

Preparation Time: 10 Minutes

Cooking Time: 1 Hour & 10 Minutes

Servings: 2

Ingredients:

- 1 cup of water
- 2 small heads of broccoli, florets
- 2 teaspoons of chopped fresh ginger
- 1 teaspoon of turmeric powder
- 1 teaspoon of salt
- 1 can of unsweetened coconut milk
- 3 cloves of garlic
- 1 onion

Directions:

1. Simmer half of the coconut milk in a skillet over low heat, then add garlic and onion.
2. Cook for around 5 minutes until they become soft. Put in the rest of the coconut milk, water, broccoli florets, ginger, turmeric, and salt, then let the mixture boil for around one hour while stirring frequently and smashing broccoli florets.
3. Leave the mix to cool before putting in a processor and processing until smooth. If

utilizing a mini processor, blend the mixture in small portions.

4. Serve with some sesame seeds, fresh greens, roasted almonds, and yogurt.

Nutrition:

Calories: 60

Carbs: 9g

Fat: 3g

Protein: 2g

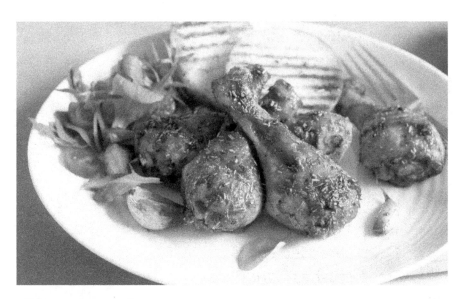

Chapter 3

Dinner

15. Keto Ham and Broccoli Creamy Casserole

Preparation time: 15 minutes

Cooking time: 45 minutes

Servings: 8

Ingredients:

- 14 oz (400g) diced ham
- 2 (14-ounce) (800g) bags frozen broccoli

- 8 oz (226g) cream cheese, softened
- 1 cup plain full-fat Greek yogurt
- ½ cup mayonnaise
- 1 tsp garlic salt
- 1 tsp onion powder
- ½ tsp dried basil
- ½ tsp smoked paprika
- ¼ tsp rosemary
- ¼ tsp thyme
- 1 cup shredded cheese
- 1 cup crushed pork rinds

Directions:

1. Prepare to preheat your oven to 350 °F (180 °C).
2. In a large bowl, add the ham, broccoli, cream cheese, yogurt, mayonnaise, garlic salt, onion powder, basil, smoked paprika, rosemary, and thyme; mix until well combined.
3. Add the casserole mixture into a greased casserole dish. Top with shredded cheese and crushed pork rinds—Bake within 45 minutes or until browned and bubbly.

Nutrition:

Calories 500

Carbs 13.6g

Fat 41.4g

Protein 42.8g

16. Chicken Skillet with Jalapeno and Cheese Sauce

Preparation time: 15 minutes

Cooking time: 25 minutes

Servings: 6

Ingredients:

- 2 tbsp olive oil
- 6 medium chicken thighs
- Salt and pepper, to taste
- ¾ tsp chili powder
- ¾ tsp cumin
- ½ cup onion, finely diced
- 3 medium jalapeños, seeds removed, finely diced
- 2 cloves garlic, minced
- ½ cup low-sodium chicken broth
- 4 oz (113g) cream cheese
- 1 cup shredded cheddar cheese

Directions:

1. Prepare to preheat your oven to 425 F and a large oven-safe skillet over medium-high heat.
2. Add one tbsp of the olive oil to the skillet. Rub over the chicken with salt, pepper, chili powder, and cumin.
3. Place the chicken in the skillet and sear on the skin side down for 8-10 minutes. Put the skillet

in the oven, then bake within 15 minutes or until cooked through.

4. Remove the chicken thighs and then drain the skillet so that only a few teaspoons of oil remain.
5. Heat the pan over medium-low heat and stir in the onion and jalapenos. Cook for about five minutes, or until softened, add the garlic and cook until fragrant.
6. Mix in the chicken broth and cream cheese. Once it turns into a cream sauce, stir in the shredded cheddar cheese. Place the chicken thighs back in the skillet, serve.

Nutrition:

Calories 279

Carbs 3.1g

Fat 22.1g

Protein 17.9g

17. Keto Creamy Sun-Dried Tomato Chicken Thighs

Preparation time: 15 minutes

Cooking time: 15 minutes

Servings: 6

Ingredients:

Chicken Thighs:

- ½ cup grated Parmesan cheese
- 6-pieces chicken thighs, skinless and boneless
- Salt and pepper, to taste

Creamy Sauce:

- ¼ cup oil from jarred sun-dried tomatoes
- 1 cup drained sun-dried tomatoes, chopped
- 4 cloves garlic, minced
- 1 tbsp Italian seasoning
- 1 cup heavy whipping cream
- ¼ cup Parmesan cheese

Directions:

1. Combine the Parmesan cheese, salt, and some pepper on a plate. Coat the chicken in the mixture evenly.
2. Warm the sun-dried tomato oil in a skillet over medium-high heat. Sear the coated chicken for a few minutes on each side, until browned. Set the seared chicken aside.

3. Place the sun-dried tomatoes, garlic, and Italian seasoning in the skillet and cook for a few minutes until the tomatoes start to soften.
4. Put in the heavy cream and the rest of the Parmesan cheese. Combine to create the finished sauce.
5. Add the seared chicken back to the skillet and cook until the chicken is cooked through.

Nutrition:

Calories 317

Carbs 8.6g

Fat 23.6g

Protein 20.3g

18. Keto Ground Beef Stroganoff

Preparation time: 15 minutes

Cooking time: 15 minutes

Servings: 4

Ingredients:

- 2 tbsp butter
- 1 clove minced garlic
- 1 pound 80% lean ground beef
- Salt and pepper, to taste
- 10 oz(228g) sliced mushrooms
- 2 tbsp water
- 1 cup sour cream
- ½ tsp paprika
- 1 tbsp fresh lemon juice
- 1 tbsp fresh chopped parsley

Directions:

1. Put the butter to dissolve in a large skillet over medium heat. When the butter has melted and stops foaming, add the minced garlic to the skillet.
2. Cook the garlic until fragrant, then mix in the ground beef—season with salt and pepper.
3. Cook the ground beef until no longer pink; break up the grounds with a wooden spoon. Remove and set aside in a bowl.
4. Leave only just a little fat in the skillet' bottom to cook the mushrooms.

5. Add the mushrooms and water to the pan and cook over medium heat. Cook until the liquid has reduced halfway, and the mushrooms are tender. Set the cooked mushrooms aside.
6. Reduce the heat, then whisk the sour cream and paprika into the skillet. Stir in the cooked beef and mushrooms into the pan and combine. Stir in the lemon juice and parsley.

Nutrition:

Calories 463

Carbs 4.1g

Fat 38.9g

Protein 23.2g

19. Keto Salisbury Steak with Mashed Cauliflower

Preparation time: 15 minutes

Cooking time: 30 minutes

Servings: 3

Ingredients:

- 3 cups cauliflower florets
- 1 tbsp butter & 1 tbsp olive oil
- 3 tbsp unsweetened almond milk
- 12 ounces ground beef
- ¼ cup almond flour
- 2 tsp fresh chopped parsley
- 2 tsp Worcestershire sauce
- ¼ tsp onion powder & ¼ tsp garlic powder
- Salt and pepper, to taste
- 1 ½ cups sliced mushrooms
- ¼ cup beef broth & 2 tbsp sour cream

Directions:

1. Boil the cauliflower in salted water within 5-8 minutes or until tender. Drain the cauliflower, add the butter and almond milk to the cauliflower mash it. Set it aside.
2. Preheat your oven to 375 °F (190 °C). Line a baking sheet with foil.
3. In a bowl, combine the ground beef, almond flour, parsley, Worcestershire sauce, onion powder, garlic powder, salt, and pepper.

4. Divide the mixture into patties and shape into the Salisbury steaks; put the patties on the foil-lined baking sheet. Bake the patties for 20 minutes or until cooked through.
5. Heat the oil in a large skillet over medium-high heat, add the mushrooms into the skillet, and then cook until they soften and brown.
6. Pour in the beef broth and stir continuously, scraping up and browned bits from the pan's bottom.
7. Stir in the sour cream, then remove the skillet from the heat—season with salt and pepper. Serve with the mashed cauliflower, drizzle with the mushroom gravy.

Nutrition:

Calories 459

Carbs 9.4g

Fat 32.3g

Protein 34.2g

20. Butter Paneer Chicken Curry

Preparation time: 15 minutes

Cooking time: 30 minutes

Servings: 5

Ingredients:

- 3 pounds bone-in chicken thighs
- 7 oz (200g) paneer packet
- 1 cup of water
- 1 cup crushed tomatoes
- ½ cup heavy whipping cream
- 4 tbsp butter
- 1 tbsp olive oil
- 2 tsp coconut oil
- 1 ½ tsp garlic paste
- 1 ½ tsp ginger paste
- 1 tsp coriander powder
- 1 tsp garam masala
- 1 tsp salt
- 1 tsp ground black pepper
- ½ tsp paprika
- ½ tsp Kashmiri Mirch
- ½ tsp red chili powder
- 5 sprigs cilantro

Directions:

1. Preheat oven to 375 °F (190 °C)
2. Rub chick thighs with olive oil, salt, and pepper to taste. Add the chicken to a baking sheet and roast for 25 minutes.
3. Slice the paneer into small pieces and set aside. Heat the butter and coconut in a pan over medium heat, let the butter start to brown.
4. Mix in the ginger plus garlic paste and sauté for 2 minutes. Add the crushed tomato to the pan.
5. Stir in the coriander powder, garam masala, paprika, red chili powder, and salt. Combine well and allow to simmer until oil shows at the top.
6. Carefully mix the paneer into the sauce. Pour in water and allow it to simmer for 5 minutes.
7. Reduce the heat to medium-low, mix the cream. Stir to combine. Let it simmer until it comes to a boil again. Separate the chicken from the bone.
8. Mix in chicken to the sauce and stir well. Let the curry simmer for at least 5 more minutes. Garnish with cilantro and serve hot.

Nutrition:

Calories 819

Carbs 3g

Fat 67.8g

Protein 50.5g

21. Pan-Seared Cod with Tomato Hollandaise

Preparation time: 15 minutes

Cooking time: 10 minutes

Servings: 4

Ingredients:

Pan-Seared Cod:

- 1 pound (4-fillets) wild Alaskan Cod
- 1 tbsp salted butter
- 1 tbsp olive oil

Tomato Hollandaise:

- 3 large egg yolks
- 3 tbsp warm water
- 226 grams salted butter, melted
- 1/4 tsp salt
- 1/4 tsp black pepper
- 2 tbsp tomato paste
- 2 tbsp fresh lemon juice

Directions:

1. Season both sides of the code fillet without salt; the salt will be added in the last. Heat a skillet over medium heat and coat with olive oil and butter.
2. When the butter heats up, place the cod fillet in the skillet and sear on both sides for 2-3

minutes. Baste the fish fillet with the oil and butter mixture.

3. You will know that the cod cooked when it flakes when poked with a fork. Melt the butter in the microwave.

4. In a double boil, beat egg yolks with warm water until thick and creamy and start forming soft peaks. Remove the double boil from the heat, gradually adding the melted butter and stirring.

5. Put salt plus pepper, stir in herbs if desired. Mix in the tomato paste. Stir to combine. Put in the lemon juice, add water to lighten the sauce texture.

Nutrition:

Calories 611

Carbs 6.9g

Fat 52g

Protein 25.8g

22. Baked Eggplant Parmesan

Preparation time: 15 minutes

Cooking time: 40 minutes

Servings: 4

Ingredients:

- 1 large eggplant, sliced into 8 1/2"
- sprinkle of salt
- 1 large egg
- ½ cup Parmesan cheese, grated
- ¼ cup ground pork rinds
- ½ tablespoon Italian seasoning
- 1 cup Rao's Arrabbiata Sauce
- ½ cup shredded mozzarella cheese
- 4 tablespoons butter melted

Directions:

1. Prepare to preheat the oven to 400 °F (200 °C). Place the eggplant slice on a baking sheet lined with baking paper and sprinkle both sides with salt. Let sit for at least 30 minutes to allow the water out.
2. Mix the ground pork rinds, parmesan cheese, and Italian seasoning in a shallow bowl. Set aside.
3. Mix the egg in a separate shallow bowl. Add the melted butter to the bottom of a 9x13 inch baking dish.
4. Pat, the eggplant dry with a kitchen towel, set aside. Dip each slice of the eggplant into the

beaten egg and then into the parmesan cheese mixture, covering each side with crumbs. Place the eggplant into the butter coated baking dish.

5. Bake the eggplants for 20 minutes. Turn the pieces over and bake an additional 20 minutes or until golden brown.
6. Pout the marinara sauce over the eggplant and sprinkle with mozzarella cheese.
7. Place the baking sheet bake in the oven for an additional 5 minutes or until the cheese has melted.

Nutrition:

Calories 313

Carbs 6.3g

Fat 25.7g

Protein 11.5g

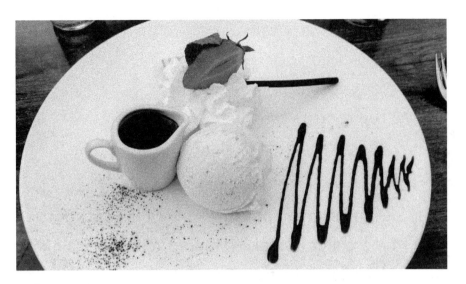

Chapter 4

Snacks

23. Yogurt with Turmeric and Coconut Cream

Preparation time: 15 minutes

Cooking time: 40 minutes

Servings: 4

Ingredients:

- 1¼ pounds of salmon
- 1 tablespoon of olive oil
- ½ cup of unsweetened grated coconut
- 1 tablespoon of turmeric

- 1 tsp of kosher salt
- ½ tsp of garlic powder
- 4 tablespoons of olive oil for frying
- 2 cup of Napa cabbage
- 1 stick of butter with salt and pepper

Directions:

1. Cut the salmon into small 1-inch pieces. Grind the coconut to make it more likely to remain in the parts of the fish.

2. If you don't have a grinder, use a sharp knife to cut the grated coconut as thin as possible. Mix the coconut powder, turmeric, salt, and garlic in a bowl. In another bowl, cover the salmon with 1 tablespoon of olive oil.

3. Take Dredge oil-coated salmon with dry ingredients—warm four tbsp of olive oil in a pan over medium heat.

4. Cook the salmon covered with coconut until it becomes crispy within one minute per side. Make sure each side is golden brown.

5. Remove and keep it warm while cooking the cabbage. Cut the cabbage into thin strips with a knife or destroy it in a food processor.

6. Melt the butter in a pan to cook the salmon. Cook the cabbage until it is tender. Season the cabbage with salt and pepper. Serve the cabbage with the salmon and enjoy

Nutrition:

Calories: 744

Carbs: 3g

Protein: 32 g

Fat: 67 g

24. Keto Tuna Casserole

Preparation time: 15 minutes

Cooking time: 30 minutes

Servings: 4

Ingredients:

- 4 spoons of Butter
- 2 spoons of olive oil
- 1 medium onion, diced
- 1 green pepper, diced
- 5 diced celery stalks
- 2 cups of finely chopped spinach
- 2 cans of tuna-in-olive oil, drained
- 1 cup of mayonnaise
- 1 ½ cup of freshly grated Parmesan
- 1 tablespoon hot pepper and salted pepper flakes

Directions:

1. Preheat the oven to 350 degrees.
2. Warm the butter plus olive oil in a large pan. Fry the onion, green pepper, celery, and spinach in the butter/oil.
3. In a bowl, mix the tuna, Parmesan, mayonnaise, and chili flakes until they are well mixed.

4. Add the sautéed vegetables to the tuna mixture and stir until everything is incorporated. Pour the tuna mixture into a pan—Bake for 30 minutes.

5. Remove the pan from the oven when it is golden brown on the top and sparkling. You can prepare the pan the day before and store it in the refrigerator.

Nutrition:

Calories: 953

Carbs: 5g

Protein: 43g

Fat: 83g

25. Cheese Stuffed Mushrooms

Preparation Time: 10 minutes

Cooking Time: 15 minutes

Servings: 12

Ingredients:

- 12 large mushrooms, clean, remove stems and chopped stems finely
- 1 ½ tbsp fresh parsley, chopped
- 4 garlic cloves, minced
- ½ cup parmesan cheese, grated
- ¼ cup Swiss cheese, grated
- 3 1/2 oz cream cheese
- 1 tbsp olive oil
- Salt

Directions:

1. Preheat the oven to 375 F.
2. Toss mushrooms with olive oil and place onto a baking tray.
3. In a bowl, combine cream cheese, chopped mushrooms stems, parsley, garlic, parmesan cheese, Swiss cheese, and salt.

4. Stuff cream cheese mixture into the mushroom caps and arrange mushrooms on the baking tray.
5. Bake in preheated oven for 10-15 minutes. Serve and enjoy.

Nutrition:

Calories 79

Fat 6.3 g

Carbs 1.5 g

Sugar 0.5 g

Protein 4 g

Cholesterol 16 mg

26. Delicious Chicken Alfredo Dip

Preparation Time: 10 minutes

Cooking Time: 20 minutes

Servings: 8

Ingredients:

- 2 cups cooked chicken, chopped
- 1 ½ tbsp fresh parsley, chopped
- 1 tomato, diced
- 2 bacon slices, cooked and crumbled
- 1 ½ cups mozzarella cheese, shredded
- 1 tsp Italian seasoning
- ½ cup parmesan cheese, grated
- 8 oz cream cheese, softened
- 1 ½ cups Alfredo sauce, homemade & low-carb

Directions:

1. Preheat the oven to 375 F.
2. Grease a baking dish using a cooking spray and set aside. Add chicken, ½ cup mozzarella cheese, Italian seasoning, parmesan cheese, cream cheese, and Alfredo sauce to the bowl and stir to combine.
3. Spread chicken mixture into the prepared baking dish and top with remaining mozzarella cheese.

4. Bake in preheated oven for 20 minutes. Top with parsley, tomatoes, and bacon. Serve and enjoy.

Nutrition:

Calories 144

Fat 0.5 g

Carbs 7.4 g

Sugar 1.3 g

Protein 29.3 g

Cholesterol 216 mg

27. Zucchini Tots

Preparation Time: 10 minutes

Cooking Time: 20 minutes

Servings: 4

Ingredients:

- 5 cups zucchini, grated and squeeze out all liquid
- ½ tsp garlic powder
- ½ tsp dried oregano
- ½ cup parmesan cheese, grated
- ½ cup cheddar cheese, shredded
- 2 eggs, lightly beaten
- Pepper
- Salt

Directions:

1. Preheat the oven to 400 F.
2. Grease a baking tray with cooking spray and set aside. Add all ingredients into the bowl and mix until well combined.
3. Make small tots from the zucchini mixture and place onto the prepared baking tray—Bake in preheated oven for 15-20 minutes. Serve and enjoy.

Nutrition:

Calories 353

Fat 23.1 g

Carbs 9.5 g

Sugar 2.8 g

Protein 32.1 g

Cholesterol 157 mg

28. Easy & Perfect Meatballs

Preparation Time: 10 minutes

Cooking Time: 20 minutes

Servings: 8

Ingredients:

- 1 egg, lightly beaten
- 3 garlic cloves, minced
- ½ cup mozzarella cheese, shredded
- ½ cup parmesan cheese, grated
- 1 lb. ground beef
- Pepper
- Salt

Directions:

1. Preheat the oven to 400 F.
2. Prepare or line a baking tray with parchment paper and set aside. Add all ingredients into the mixing bowl and mix until well combined.
3. Make small balls from meat mixture and place on a prepared baking tray—Bake in preheated oven for 20 minutes. Serve and enjoy.

Nutrition:

Calories 157

Fat 6.7 g

Carbs 0.5 g

Protein21.5 g

Sugar 0.1 g

Cholesterol 80mg

29. Eggplant Chips

Preparation Time: 10 minutes

Cooking Time: 20 minutes

Servings: 15

Ingredients:

- 1 large eggplant, thinly sliced
- ¼ cup parmesan cheese, grated
- 1 tsp dried oregano
- ¼ tsp dried basil
- ½ tsp garlic powder
- ¼ cup olive oil
- ¼ tsp pepper
- ½ tsp salt

Directions:

1. Preheat the oven to 325 F.
2. In a small bowl, mix oil and dried spices.
3. Coat eggplant with oil and spice mixture and arrange eggplant slices on a baking tray—Bake in preheated oven for 15-20 minutes. Turn halfway through.
4. Remove from oven and sprinkle with grated cheese. Serve and enjoy.

Nutrition:

Calories 77

Fat 5.8 g

Carbs 2 g

Protein 3.5 g

Sugar 0.9 g

Cholesterol 8mg

30. Healthy Chicken Fritters

Preparation Time: 10 minutes

Cooking Time: 20 minutes

Servings: 4

Ingredients:

- 1 ½ lb. chicken breast, skinless, boneless, and chopped into small pieces
- 1 tbsp olive oil
- ½ tsp garlic powder
- 2 tbsp fresh parsley, chopped
- 1 ½ tbsp chives, chopped
- 1 ½ tbsp fresh basil, chopped
- 1 cup mozzarella cheese, shredded
- 1/3 cup almond flour
- 2 eggs, lightly beaten
- Pepper
- Salt

Directions:

1. Add all ingredients except oil into the large mixing bowl and mix until well combined.
2. Heat oil in a pan over medium heat. Scoop fritter mixture using a large spoon and transfer

it to the pan and cook for 6-8 minutes or until golden brown on both sides. Serve and enjoy.

Nutrition:

Calories 331

Fat 15.9 g

Carbs 2.9 g

Protein 43 g

Sugar 0.6 g

Cholesterol 194mg

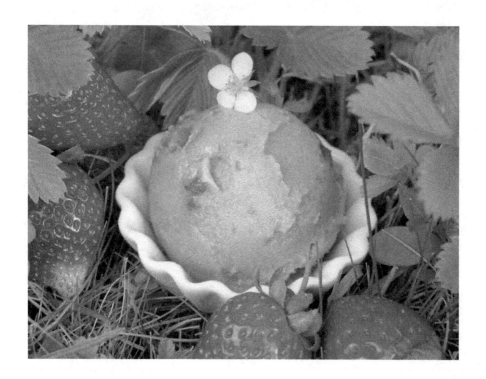

Chapter 5

Dessert

31. Vanilla Cupcakes

Preparation time: 15 minutes

Cooking time: 30 minutes

Servings: 32

Ingredients:

- 1 cup almond milk, unsweetened

- 1 cup almond flour
- ¾ cup erythritol, powdered
- ½ cup butter
- 7 eggs
- 1 tablespoon baking powder
- 3 teaspoons vanilla extract
- ½ teaspoon liquid stevia
- Salt

Directions:

1. Preheat the oven to 350 F.
2. Pour the batter into cupcake liners, then bake them for 28 to 30 mins. Allow the cupcakes to cool, then serve them with your favorite toppings and enjoy.

Nutrition:

Calories: 100

Fat: 7.1 g

Protein: 2.1 g

Carbs: 8 g

32. Cocoa Mocha Truffles

Preparation time: 15 minutes

Cooking time: 0 minutes

Servings: 15 to 20

Ingredients:

- 7 ounces butter, unsalted
- 4 tablespoons strong brewed coffee
- 2 tablespoons honey
- 2 tablespoons cocoa powder
- ½ teaspoon vanilla powder
- ½ teaspoon cinnamon
- Salt

Directions:

1. Spoon two teaspoons of the mix, shape it into balls, roll them in some cocoa powder or chopped nuts.
2. Repeat the process with the remaining mix, freeze them for 1 hour, then serve them and enjoy.

Nutrition:

Calories: 93

Fat: 9.6 g

Protein: 0.2 g

Carbs: 2.5 g

33. Vanilla Ice Cream

Preparation time: 20 minutes

Cooking time: 0 minutes

Servings: 6

Ingredients:

- 4 egg whites
- 4 egg yolks
- 1 ¼ cup heavy whipping cream
- ½ cup erythritol, powdered
- 1 tablespoon vanilla extract
- ¼ teaspoon cream of tartar

Directions:

1. Whisk the whipped cream in another bowl until it's soft peaks. Whisk the egg yolks until they become pale, then add the vanilla and whisk them again.
2. Spoon the mix into a loaf pan and freeze it for 2 hours, then serve your ice cream and enjoy it.

Nutrition:

Calories: 226

Fat: 12.3 g

Protein: 4.8 g

Carbs: 24.9 g

34. Snow Bites

Preparation time: 20 minutes

Cooking time: 18 minutes

Servings: 36

Ingredients:

- 2 cups almond flour
- 1 cup walnuts, finely chopped
- ¾ and ½ cup erythritol, powdered
- ½ cup butter softened
- 1 egg
- 2 tablespoons coconut flour
- 1 teaspoon vanilla extract
- 1 teaspoon baking powder
- ¾ teaspoon cardamom powder
- ¼ teaspoon Stevia extract
- Salt

Directions:

1. Preheat the oven to 325 F.
2. Mix the cardamom powder with a pinch of salt, coconut flour, walnut, baking powder, and almond flour in a mixing bowl.
3. Beat ½ cup of erythritol with butter in a mixing bowl until it becomes light and fluffy, then add the egg with stevia and vanilla and beat them again.

4. Add the almond mix to the butter and mix them until they make a smooth dough, then shape it into ¾ inch balls.
5. Place the dough balls on two lined baking sheets and bake them for 18 mins.
6. Once the time is up, toss the almond balls in a large bowl gently with ¾ cup of erythritol until coated, then serve them and enjoy.

Nutrition:

Calories: 40

Fat: 7.4 g

Protein: 2.1 g

Carbs: 5.5 g

35. Blueberry Ice Cream

Preparation time: 15 minutes

Cooking time: 0 minutes

Servings: 4

Ingredients:

- 1 cup heavy whipping cream
- ½ cup crème Fraiche
- ½ cup blueberries
- 2 egg yolks
- 1 tablespoon vanilla powder

Directions:

1. Whip the whipping cream until it becomes fluffy, then set it aside.
2. Beat the crème Fraiche until it becomes fluffy, then add the whipping cream, vanilla, blueberries, and egg yolks and beat them again until they become creamy.
3. Spoon the ice cream into a loaf pan and freeze it for 1 hour, then serve it and enjoy it.

Nutrition:

Calories: 202

Fat: 19 g

Protein: 2.4 g

Carbs: 4.6 g

36. Pecan Pie Ice Cream

Preparation time: 15 minutes

Cooking time: 0 minutes

Servings: 4

Ingredients:

- 2 cups of coconut milk
- ½ cup pumpkin purée
- ½ cup cottage cheese
- ½ cup pecans, toasted and chopped
- 1/3 cup erythritol, powdered
- 3 egg yolks
- 20 drops liquid Stevia
- 1 teaspoon pumpkin spice
- 1 teaspoon maple extract
- ½ teaspoon xanthan gum powder

Directions:

1. Blend them with an immersion blender until they become smooth.
2. Pour the mix into an ice cream machine, stir in the toasted pecans, and then prepare it according to the manufacturer's instructions.
3. Serve your ice cream and enjoy it.

Nutrition:

Calories: 467

Fat: 37.2 g

Protein: 6 g

Carbs: 34.3 g

37. Chocolate Bites

Preparation time: 20 minutes

Cooking time: 20 minutes

Servings: 20

Ingredients:

- 1 cup almond flour
- 1/3 cup coconut, shredded
- 1/3 cup erythritol, powdered
- ¼ cup of coconut oil
- ¼ cup of cocoa powder
- 2 eggs
- 3 tablespoons coconut flour
- 1 teaspoon vanilla extract
- ½ teaspoon baking powder
- Salt

Directions:

1. Preheat the oven to 350 F.
2. Mix the shredded coconut and coconut flour with cocoa powder, erythritol, almond flour, baking powder, and a pinch of salt in a large bowl.
3. Add the vanilla with coconut oil and eggs, then knead them to get a smooth dough.

4. Shape the dough into 20 balls, then place them on a lined baking sheet and bake them for 15 to 20 mins. Once the time is up, serve your chocolate bites and enjoy it.

Nutrition:

Calories: 85

Fat: 6.4 g

Protein: 1.9 g

Carbs: 6.7 g

38. Swiss Roll

Preparation time: 25 minutes

Cooking time: 15 minutes

Servings:12

Ingredients:

- 8 ounces cream cheese
- 1 cup almond flour
- ½ cup erythritol, powder
- ½ cup sour cream
- ¼ cup of cocoa powder
- ¼ cup of coconut milk
- ¼ cup psyllium husk powder
- 12 tablespoons butter
- 3 eggs
- 2 teaspoons vanilla extract
- 1 teaspoon baking powder
- ¼ teaspoon liquid Stevia
- Salt

Directions:

1. Mix the almond flour with ¼ cup of cocoa powder, psyllium husk powder, baking powder, ¼ cup of erythritol, and a pinch of salt in a large mixing bowl.
2. Add in 4 tablespoons of butter with coconut milk, ¼ cup of sour cream, eggs, and one teaspoon of vanilla extract and mix them again until they become smooth.

3. Prepare to preheat the oven to 350 F. Transfer the mix to a lined baking sheet and press it to make the crust, then bake it for 12 to 15 mins.
4. Beat the remaining eight tablespoons of butter with ¼ cup of erythritol, one teaspoon of vanilla, stevia, ¼ cup of sour cream, and cream cheese until they become light and fluffy to make the filling.
5. Put the filling all over the crust and roll it gently. Serve your Swiss Roll with your favorite toppings and enjoy.

Nutrition:

Calories: 274.2

Fat: 25.1 g

Protein: 5.3 g

Carbs: 6.8 g

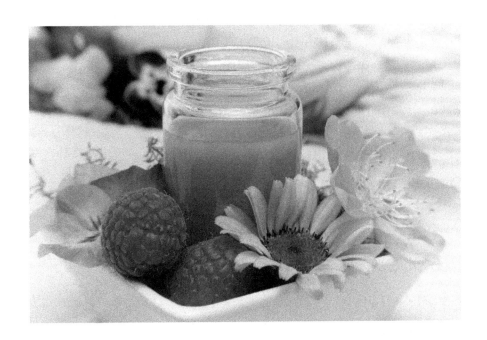

Chapter 6

Smoothies

39. Lemony Green Smoothie

Preparation Time: 10 minutes

Cooking time: 0 minutes

Servings: 2

Ingredients:

- 2 large green apples, cored and sliced

- 4 cups fresh kale leaves
- 4 tablespoons fresh parsley leaves
- 1 tablespoon fresh ginger, peeled
- 1 lemon, peeled
- ½ cup of filtered water
- Pinch of salt

Directions:

1. Place all the fixing in a blender and pulse until well combined. Strain and serve immediately.

Nutrition:

Calories: 196

Sodium: 21 mg

Fiber: 1.4 g

Fat: 1.1 g

Carbs: 1.6 g

Protein: 1.5 g

40. Berry Soy Yogurt Parfait

Preparation Time: 2-4 minutes

Cooking time: 0 minute

Servings: 1

Ingredients:

- 1 carton vanilla cultured soy yogurt
- 1/4 cup granola (gluten-free)
- 1 cup berries (you can take strawberries, blueberries, raspberries, blackberries)

Directions:

1. Put half of the yogurt in a glass jar or serving dish. On the top, put half of the berries.
2. Then sprinkle with half of the granola—repeat layers. Serve.

Nutrition:

Calories: 244,

Sodium: 33 mg,

Fiber: 1.4 g,

Fat: 3.1 g,

Carbs: 11.3 g,

Protein: 1.4 g.

41. Orange & Celery Crush

Preparation Time: 10 minutes

Cooking Time: 0 minutes

Servings: 1

Ingredients:

- 1 carrot, peeled
- Stalks of celery
- 1 orange, peeled
- ½ teaspoon matcha powder
- Juice of 1 lime

Directions:

1. Place ingredients into a blender with enough water to cover them and blitz until smooth.

Nutrition:

Calories: 150

Sodium: 31 mg

Fiber: 1.2 g

Fat: 2.1 g

Carbs: 11.2 g

Protein: 1.4 g

42. Creamy Strawberry & Cherry Smoothie

Preparation Time: 10 minutes

Cooking Time: 0 minutes

Servings: 1

Ingredients:

- 3½ ounce. Strawberries
- 3 1/2 ounce of frozen pitted cherries
- 1 tablespoon plain full-fat yogurt
- 6 1/2 ounce of unsweetened soya milk

Directions:

1. Place the ingredients into a blender, then process until smooth. Serve and enjoy.

Nutrition:

Calories: 203

Sodium: 23 mg

Fiber: 1.4 g

Fat: 3.1 g

Carbs: 12.3 g

Protein: 1.7 g

43. Grapefruit & Celery Blast

Preparation Time: 10 minutes

Cooking Time: 0 minutes

Servings: 1

Ingredients

- 1 grapefruit, peeled
- stalks of celery
- 2-ounce kale
- ½ teaspoon matcha powder

Directions:

1. Place ingredients into a blender with water to cover them and blitz until smooth.

Nutrition:

Calories: 129

Sodium: 24 mg

Fiber: 1.4 g

Fat: 2.1 g

Carbs: 12.1 g

Protein: 1.2 g

44. Walnut & Spiced Apple Tonic

Preparation Time: 10 minutes

Cooking Time: 0 minutes

Servings: 1

Ingredients:

- 6 walnuts halves
- 1 apple, cored
- 1 banana
- ½ teaspoon matcha powder
- ½ teaspoon cinnamon
- Pinch of ground nutmeg

Directions:

1. Place ingredients into a blender and add sufficient water to cover them. Blitz until smooth and creamy.

Nutrition:

Calories: 124

Sodium: 22 mg

Fiber: 1.4 g

Fat: 2.1 g

Carbs: 12.3 g

Protein: 1.2 g

45. Tropical Chocolate Delight

Preparation Time: 10 minutes

Cooking Time: 0 minutes

Servings: 1

Ingredients:

- 1 mango, peeled & de-stoned
- ounce fresh pineapple, chopped
- 2 ounces of kale
- 1 ounce of rocket
- 1 tablespoon 100% cocoa powder or cacao nibs
- 1 ounce of coconut milk

Direction

1. Place ingredients into a blender and blitz until smooth. You can add a little water if it seems too thick.

Nutrition:

Calories: 192

Sodium: 26 mg

Fiber: 1.3 g

Fat: 4.1 g

Carbs: 16.6 g

Protein: 1.6 g

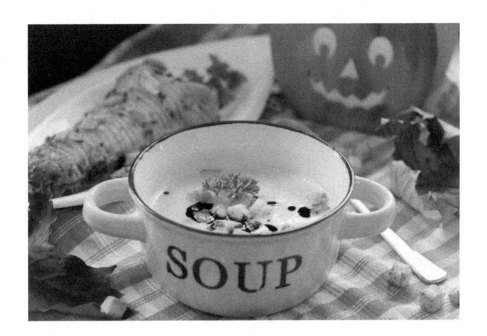

Chapter 7

Soups

46. Cream of Asparagus Soup

Preparation time: 15 minutes

Cooking time: 23 minutes

Servings: 2

Ingredients:

- 2 cups reduced-sodium chicken broth
- 1 tablespoon unsalted butter

- ¾ pound asparagus, cut in half
- Salt and black pepper, to taste
- 3 tablespoons sour cream

Directions:

1. Warm-up butter in a large pot over medium-low heat and add asparagus. Sauté for about 3 minutes and stir in the chicken broth, salt, and black pepper.
2. Bring to a boil, cover, and cook for about 20 minutes on low heat. Remove from heat and transfer into a blender along with sour cream.
3. Pulse until smooth and spoon out in a bowl to serve.

Nutrition:

Calories 140

Fat 9.7g

Cholesterol 23mg

Sodium 686mg

Carbs 8.3g

Fiber 3.6g

Sugars 3.8g

Protein 7.6g

47. French Onion Soup

Preparation time: 15 minutes

Cooking time: 35 minutes

Servings: 2

Ingredients:

- 1/3-pound brown onions

- 1 tablespoon butter

- 2 drops liquid Stevia

- 1½ cups beef stock

- 1 tablespoon olive oil

Directions:

1. Warm-up butter and olive oil in a large pot over medium-low heat and add onions.

2. Sauté for about 4 minutes and stir in beef stock and stevia. Cook for about 5 minutes and reduce the heat to low.

3. Allow to simmer for about 25 minutes and ladle out into soup bowls to serve hot.

Nutrition:

Calories 152

Fat 13.2g

Cholesterol 15mg

Sodium 533mg

Carbs 7.1g

Fiber 1.6g

Sugars 3.2g

Protein 2.6g

48. Green Chicken Enchilada Soup

Preparation time: 15 minutes

Cooking time: 5 minutes

Servings: 2

Ingredients:

- ¼ cup salsa Verde
- 2 oz. cream cheese softened
- ½ cup cheddar cheese, shredded
- 1½ cups chicken stock
- 1 cup cooked chicken, shredded

Directions:

1. Put cheddar cheese, salsa Verde, cream cheese, and chicken stock in an immersion blender.
2. Blend until smooth and pour this mixture into a medium saucepan. Cook for about 5 minutes on medium heat and add the shredded chicken.
3. Cook for another 5 minutes and dish out into a bowl to serve hot.

Nutrition:

Calories 333

Fat 219g

Cholesterol 115mg

Sodium 1048mg

Carbs 3g

Fiber 0.1g

Sugars 1.2g

Protein 30.4g

49. Cheesy Mushroom Shrimp Soup

Preparation time: 15 minutes

Cooking time: 15 minutes

Servings: 2

Ingredients:

- 6 oz. extra small shrimp

- 2 oz cheddar cheese, shredded

- ½ cup mushrooms, sliced

- ¼ cup butter

- 12 oz. chicken broth

Directions:

1. Put chicken broth and mushrooms in a soup pot and bring to a boil. Lower the heat and stir in butter and cheddar cheese.

2. Mix well and add shrimp to the soup pot. Allow it to simmer for about 15 minutes and dish out into a bowl to serve hot.

Nutrition:

Calories 454

Fat 34.9g

Cholesterol 271mg

Sodium 1684mg

Carbs 3.1g

Fiber 0.2g

Sugars 1g

Protein 30.8g

50. Bacon and Pumpkin Soup

Preparation time: 15 minutes

Cooking time: 8 hours & 5 minutes

Servings: 2

Ingredients:

- 1½ cups bacon hock, diced
- 100g pumpkin, diced
- Boiling water
- Salt, to taste
- 1 tablespoon butter

Directions:

1. Pour some boiling water into the slow cooker. Add pumpkin and bacon hock and cover the lid.
2. Cook on low for about 8 hours and pull the meat away from the bones. Return the meat to the slow cooker along with salt and butter.
3. Allow it to simmer for about 5 minutes and spoon out into a bowl to serve hot.

Nutrition:

Calories 286

Fat 16.5g

Cholesterol 108mg

Sodium 186mg

Carbs 4.1g

Fiber 1.5g

Sugars 1.7g

Protein 9.2g

51. Mint Avocado Chilled Soup

Preparation time: 15 minutes

Cooking time: 0 minutes

Servings: 2

Ingredients:

- 1 medium ripe avocado
- 2 romaine lettuce leaves
- 1 cup coconut milk, chilled
- Salt, to taste
- 20 fresh mint leaves

Directions:

1. Put mint leaves with the rest of the ingredients in a blender and blend until smooth.
2. Refrigerate for about 20 minutes and remove to serve chilled.

Nutrition:

Calories 309

Fat 31.2g

Cholesterol 0mg

Sodium 99mg

Carbs 9.1g

Fiber 4.9g

Sugars 4.1g

Protein 3.6g

Conclusion

Congratulations on making it through this part! It only means that you have greatly impacted your healthy lifestyle as a woman after her 50's by gaining all the knowledge about Keto Diet and how you can benefit from it.

Many women want to lose weight, but women over the age of 50 are particularly interested in losing weight, boosting their immune system, and having more energy.

If you fit into this group, this last part of this guide will address the particular hurdles you may face when doing the Keto diet. For one thing, women in this age range experience slowing metabolisms, making it harder to drop pounds than ever before.

We will cover the tweaks you can make to your Keto diet and lifestyle to accommodate these particular hurdles. We will talk about any concerns you may have and give you solutions to counteract them.

Women go through menopause sometime between the ages of 45 and 55, which can be a particularly difficult time. They notice they are putting on weight, and they experience all kinds of unpleasant symptoms such as difficulty sleeping and hot flashes.

But many of these symptoms are temporary. The one that bothers women the most is the one that lasts: weight gain. Women over 50 want to know how they can stave off weight gain and lose the extra pounds they started to put on after menopause.

Women in this age range can still go wrong when they try Keto and autophagy, so we have some pieces of advice to give you if you count yourself among this group.

The first piece of advice is to make sure you eat enough protein every day. You might be worried about eating too much protein because you are watching calories, which is a reasonable thing to do. But when you are on Keto, you need protein as a source of energy.

It is always about balance. On the one hand, you need to make up for the energy you won't be getting from carbs. On the other hand, you have to be careful not to eat too many calories.

As usual, follow along with what your body is telling you. If your body tells you that you still need more energy, wait a bit. You can eat more if some time passes and you still feel hungry. That probably means you need energy food. But you have to give yourself this waiting period because otherwise, your mind might be trying to trick you into just eating something you are craving when you are not genuinely hungry.

There is a mental component to this change in diet, too. The problem at the center of women not being able to change their diet is not being used to the real feeling of being full. By the "real" feeling of being full, we refer to how people feel when they have eaten enough—not too much.

These days, people eat so many carbs that their idea of fullness is the uncomfortable feeling when they eat too many carbs. But you can't lose weight if you see fullness this way. You will consistently overstuff yourself, believing you are making yourself full when you are gorging yourself.

To remind yourself what fullness feels like, get used to eating without overstuffing yourself. Get used to not feel uncomfortable after eating. It can feel strangely comforting to be overstuffed with carbs, but that is not a feeling we can let ourselves get used to. If we do, we will never be happy with the simple feeling of fullness.

As we keep emphasizing, we can't villainize fat anymore. The real problem is eating too many calories, most of which tend to come from carbs, not fats. However, in particular, women over 50 need to be careful not to eat too many fats when they follow Keto.

Keto isn't a valid excuse for simply eating a ton of fat. You still need to show some constraint as you do in every diet. Understanding how to balance your fat consumption will take learning how fat fits into Keto. With Keto, you want to be what we call fat-adapted.

You already know what this means; it is just another way of saying what happens in Ketosis. Being fat-adapted means you are burning fat for energy with Ketones instead of burning glucose with carbs.

We tell you this term because you should eat many healthy fats until you go through significant Ketosis—until you are fat-adapted. Once that happens, you should start being more careful with how much fat you are consuming.

One of the sources women over 50 will get fat from is drinks. Even the drinks you make at home, like coffee with milk, can be a lot higher in fat than you think. It should go without saying that the specialty coffee you get topped with whipped cream is high in fat.

Women over 50 know they have their hurdles to overcome when they chase weight loss goals and improve overall health with Keto. But they can do all they can do by following along with the advice in this guide. So, all in all, you have nothing to worry about! We've got your back. Happy-healthy eating!

CPSIA information can be obtained
at www.ICGtesting.com
Printed in the USA
BVHW041622300421
606221BV00014B/2068